SPINES OF STEEL, GOLD AND RUBBER

How the Medical Profession Has Prostituted Itself For the Medical Industrial Complex

William A. Stewart, M.D.

FOREWORD

America has the best medical care in the world available in some of our major medical centers and private clinics. The constant stream of patients to these centers from all corners of the globe bears witness to this excellent level of care, including spine surgery, which is the subject of this attempt at Swiftian humor to draw attention to a nationwide problem of too much of the wrong type or unnecessary spine surgery. One need only read the periodic reports in the national press of ongoing disasters affecting large numbers of patients stemming from an out of control spine surgeon to realize the seriousness of this problem.

Equally disturbing is the failure of the various state licensing boards and professional organizations to effectively monitor spine surgeons and hospital administrators who overlook substandard medical care in an effort to increase their organization's income.

W. A. Stewart, M.D.

AUTHOR'S DISCLAIMER

This is a work of fiction. Names, characters and incidents are either products of the author's imagination or are used facetiously. Any resemblance to actual events or locales or persons living or dead, is entirely coincidental.

ABOUT THE AUTHOR

Dr. William Stewart received his M.D. from the Ohio State University College of Medicine. He completed his general surgery and neurosurgery residency training, in addition to a two-year research fellowship. He was a member of the American Association of Neurological Surgeons, the Society of Medical Consultants to the Armed Forces, and a Fellow of the American College of Surgeons, among numerous other professional organizations.

He is retired USNR and spent his activity duty as a surgeon with the Marines in Vietnam. During the Soviet invasion of Afghanistan he worked in the Mujahedeen field hospitals. He spent a year as Director of a Project Hope mission in West Africa.

Until recently he was a Professor of Clinical Neurosurgery.

RECOGNITION

I am grateful to the following individuals for their help and advice, without which the composition of this satire would not have been possible. My sincerest thanks to Suzanne, Cathleen, Sarah, Nancy, Alexandra, Joan and Michele.

CAST OF CHARACTERS

Administration, New Age Medical Center (NAMC)

President: Dr. P. H. Narrsey
Dean: Dr. D.B.L. Zero
C.E.O.:   Dr. E.D. Shiftworkski
CFO: Attorney Rele Slymowicz

Department of Neurosurgery, New Age Medical Center

Chairman: Dr. C. H. Querbol
Complex Spine Surgeon: Dr. Mick MacBuckmaker
Staff: Dr. W. B. Suum
Staff: Dr. O. O. Seven

Faculty, New Age Medical Center

Chair, Medical Complications Committee: Dr. Williams
Medical Complications Committee: Ms. Able, R.N.
                                          Ms. Baker, R.N.
                                          Dr. Snow Queen
                                          Dr. Nicodeum
Endoscopic Department: Dr. Jones
Imaging Department: Dr. R. R. Rad
                                          Dr. Excel
Director, One Day Surgery Center: Dr. Charles

Physicians Monitoring Committee (PMC)

Chairman: Dr. Jeckel
Council: Attorney Ducus
Regional Investigator: Ms. Delta

Additional Organizations

National Medical Center Review Board (NMCRB)
Physicians' Protection Program (PPP)
North Kompliant Review Board (NKRB)

CONTENTS

I.   Executive Committee Meeting, New Age Medical
        Center (NAMC)

II.   Medical Complications Committee, NAMC, One Year
        Later

III.   Executive Committee, NAMC, Six Months Later

IV.   National Medical Center Review Board (NMCRB)
        Interview, One Week Later

V.   Medical Complications Committee,
        Three Months Later

VI.   Executive Committee, NAMC, One Month Later

VII.   President Narrsey's Large, Cherry Paneled Office,
        One Month Later

VIII.   Physicians Monitoring Committee (PMC)
        Commissioner's Office, Two Months Later

IX.   Executive Committee, NAMC, One Month Later

X.   Regional PMC Investigative Office, One Month Later

XI.   Executive Committee, NAMC, Two Months Later

XII.   PMC Commissioner's Office, Three Months Later

XIII.   President Narrsey's Large, Cherry Paneled Office,
        NAMC, One Week Later

XIV.   Spine Surgery Office, NAMC, One Week Later

XV.   Office of Attorney T. K. Boutique, One Day Later

XVI.   Executive Committee, NAMC, One Week Later

XVII. Neurosurgery Clinic, NAMC, One Week Later

XVIII. PMC Central Office, One Month Later

XIX.   President Narrsey's Large, Cherry Paneled Office,
       One Month later

XX.   PMC Central Office, Two Weeks Later

XXI.   President Narrsey's Large, Cherry Paneled Office

I.

Executive Committee, New Age Medical Center (NAMC)

It is not the man who has too little, but the man who craves more, that is poor.

~Seneca

Year One

"I am going to squeeze Mercy Hospital dry and ruin them, after which I'll take them over for peanuts rather than the reasonable offer they have refused."

With these words Dr. P.H. Narrsey, President of the New Age Medical Center, vented his fury at his failed first attempt to incorporate the other hospitals in the city into his vision of a super-regional medical center that would dominate and control every aspect of health care in the western half of the state of New Amsterdam.

President Narrsey was not a force to be taken lightly. Ivy educated, confident of his viewpoints, slim, above average height with a carefully waxed handlebar mustache, he was quick to silence any opinions that were counter to his. Several former faculty members had learned this the hard way after questioning his decisions.

The last item on the agenda that day was a recommendation from the Chief Financial Officer of the medical center to change operating room procedures. This change, which had been suggested by the spine surgery service, would significantly increase revenue generated by the spine surgeons and thus increase income for the medical center administration.

A percentage of each department's income went to the administration for operating expenses. CFO Rele Slymowicz was an attorney by education who never overlooked a way to pad the bottom line of a financial report. Gruff, overweight, unconcerned about his appearance, he was aggressive in pushing his viewpoint and in personal confrontations deferred only to President Narrsey.

The CFO began his presentation by summarizing a recent meeting with the spine surgeon, Dr. Mick MacBuckmaker. According to Dr. MacBuckmaker over the past several years, thanks to advances in the specialty of complex spine surgery, the volume of this type of surgery had exploded across the country. Political maneuvering by the medical industrial complex which made the hardware for these procedures had enabled fees for these operations to increase exponentially.

For example, where formerly a simple one-level herniated disc was treated by a partial hemi-laminectomy and excision of the disc for $1,000, it was now accepted practice to treat the same condition with a two- or three-level fusion for $15,000. Furthermore, the indications for surgery had become so relaxed that many more complaints, even back and neck pain alone, were now considered indications for fusion.

Dr. MacBuckmaker proclaimed that in his opinion, any patient referred to him was fair game for a fusion, since that is what he did and the referring physician should know that.

The CFO continued, "In certain areas fees well over $100,000 are deemed reasonable and are realized for fusions. Less ambitious surgeons have morphed into one-trick ponies, giving up emergency call, and doing only small fusions in outpatient surgery centers."

Slymowicz was aware, but did not mention, that MacBuckmaker was building a multi-million dollar house on the shore, owned two Mercedes and a Lamborghini, and had ordered a large yacht built in Holland to be delivered the following year.

The CFO had also reviewed the financial statements from the spine surgery department, which was more than enough information to convince him that complex spine surgery was a cash cow. Dr. MacBuckmaker's proposal had fallen on fertile ground and Slymowicz had therefore put it on today's agenda.

With this introduction, CFO Slymowicz outlined a scheme to double the number of complex spine surgeries at University Hospital and thus increase by 100 per cent the income from the spine surgery department to the administration. Rather than have all complex spine surgery done by Dr. MacBuckmaker, who was the only one in the department certified to do these procedures, two cases would be scheduled simultaneously. MacBuckmaker would do the instrumentation in each case, but another surgeon would do the opening and closing. Mr. Slymowicz pointed out with great enthusiasm that rather than doing two or three cases a day, as many as six a day could be done for an additional tens of thousands of dollars in income.

The CFO sat back, satisfied that his proposal would meet with the committee's approval. His confidence was bolstered by the fact that President Narrsey had already given his enthusiastic agreement. A few long seconds passed before other members of the committee raised questions.

"Would this comply with regulations set forth by the State Office of Physician Monitoring?" asked Dr. Williams.

"Would this crowd out operating time for other types of surgery since we know the OR is already fully booked most of the time?" wondered Dr. Jones.

"Can you be sure there are legitimate indications for all of these complex spine surgeries?" questioned Dr. Nicodeum.

CFO Slymowicz became visibly agitated as the committee brought forth question after question, raising troublesome

3

inquiries over his planned expansion of medical center income. Finally Dr. W. B. Suum voiced an objection that should have terminated the plan then and there. Suum, a member of Dr. MacBuckmaker's department, pointed out that unexpected complications and delays would make it impossible to time the placement of instrumentation in the middle of each case, and as a result MacBuckmaker would not always be available as needed. This could cause unacceptable delays in surgery and even situations where the uncertified surgeon with a resident would be required to do the complex part of the case.

At this, Slymowicz went into a ranting frenzy; pushing away from the table, splashing coffee as he arose from his chair to pace around the room glowering at this inquisitors.

"Suum, do you think that the pennies you bring in from your pediatric surgery practice do anything significant for this institution? The income your puny practice provides would not pay the liquor bill for the appreciation dinner we put on for high rollers last month, which earned us $2,000,000 in donations for the building fund!

"Williams, you're so engrossed in researching one muscle in the left eye it is a mystery to me how you find your way to this meeting from your rat hole hospital office. You are so out of it, your wife not only has to pack your lunch for you, she has to come to your office every noon and feed it to you. Nicodeum, your ethical concepts are thousands of years behind the times. The NAMC represents the best in up-to-date, progressive thinking and our programs must be funded. And they will be - with or without your approval.

"Jones, how does someone like you, peering up people's asses in the endoscopic suite all day, think you can comment on what goes on in the main OR where the big bucks are generated?"

Slymowicz continued, his face flushed with anger, "I've spent days putting this plan together, and it is brilliant!" His voice rose in frustration. "Why are you always raising objections when I try to get this place to turn a profit? Do you have any idea how much money we are talking about? Do you actually want to make less money?" Crimson faced and shouting, he concluded, "What is wrong with you people?"

CFO Slymowicz turned to President Narrsey and blurted out his request that the committee's questions be terminated because everyone was obviously missing the point of the proposal and that Dr. MacBuckmaker be allowed to proceed in double-time with what he was doing so well - turning a profit.

The president surveyed the room, touched his mustache with his right hand, and terminated the meeting with a declaration that Slymowicz's requests were in the best interest of the medical center. He then invited everyone to join him in his large, cherry paneled office for wine and oatmeal raisin cookies.

II.

Medical Complications Committee, NAMC

It made our hair stand up in panic and fear.

~Euripides

One year later

"Have you double checked these mortality and infection rates for the spine surgery service?" asked Dr. Williams, Chairman of the Medical Complications Committee, looking in disbelief at the reports submitted by nurse practitioners Able and Baker.

"Yes, three times actually," replied Ms. Able as Ms. Baker nodded her head in agreement.

"Five times the expected mortality and infection rate when compared with the data from 150 other academic hospitals in the country!" exclaimed Dr. Williams. He made a note to himself to bring this problem up at the next Executive Committee meeting.

Dr. Jones from the Endoscopic Department asked if the past year's rates were associated with any other variables observed during this period.

"Well," commented Ms. Able, "the number of complex spine surgeries has doubled during the past year."

"That's interesting," remarked Williams, recalling the contentious Executive Committee Meeting he had attended a year ago.

"Furthermore," offered Ms. Baker, "this puts the NAMC dead last in these categories for all the academic centers doing complex spine surgery."

Dr. Jones volunteered that the term 'dead' took on additional significance in this situation, his black humor evoking a few grimaces around the table.

"Just one more matter to consider and we'll be done for today." said Dr. Williams, as he distributed the report on urinary tract infections in catheterized patients to the committee. "This rate is unacceptable. And significantly higher than past years." he added as he glanced over the table at Ms. Able and Ms. Baker. "How can this be explained?"

"The explanation seems obvious to us." replied Ms. Baker, as Ms. Able nodded in agreement. "Remember the policy implemented by Slymowicz last year in which insertion of catheters and their care is to be done by student volunteers, rather than by nursing staff?" This in turn had permitted some high salaried nurses to be terminated, allegedly without a decrease in hospital services.

Dr. Jones remembered that discussion in great detail. Because of the decrease in state financial aid the decision had been made to terminate some nursing staff, rather than decrease the number of administrative personnel at the medical center.

III.

Executive Committee, NAMC

Oh what a tangled web we weave when first we practice to deceive.

~Sir Walter Scott

Six months later

Committee members took their seats around the table as they speculated to each other about why President Narrsey had called an emergency meeting with just one hour's notice. As the last member took her seat, the President entered the room from his large, cherry paneled office, accompanied by his favorite department chair, Professor Snow Queen. He was obviously upset.

"An unscheduled review of the medical center will take place next week by the National Medical Center Review Board (NMCRB) as a consequence of reports to that body by unknown hospital employees. I assure you that I will personally see to it that the as yet unknown 'snitches' are appropriately dealt with."

"Next," he coldly proclaimed, "we must devise a plan to divert and mitigate the allegations that have been made, since we cannot afford a probation or suspension decision from the NMCRB."

Glancing over the gathered committee members, he said, "First, how do we explain or mitigate the report that Dr. MacBuckmaker dictated an operative note for a patient he did not operate on and for which he billed the patient?"

Dr. W. B. Suum immediately replied, "We don't explain it." "It's unethical 'ghost surgery'. It's happening because of your CFO's policy to double book spinal fusion cases, and it should be stopped. Now."

CFO Slymowicz immediately took the floor. "This is a matter with legal implications, and I will handle it appropriately during the NMCRB query."

President Narrsey, himself an expert in ingratiating himself and pulling the wool over the eyes of others, replied, "I trust you to do just that, Slymowicz, but there is still more to the investigation than allegations of 'ghost surgery'. For instance, Professor Querbol, chairman of MacBuckmaker's department, is not only involved in the 'ghost surgery' case, since he was the other surgeon doing the opening and closing of MacBuckmaker's surgeries, but he has also been reported for falsifying histories and physical exams for patients he was operating on in the same-day surgery clinic."

Again, CFO Slymowicz took the floor. "Have these alleged medical indiscretions been videotaped? If not, nothing can be proved."

Dr. Charles, Director of the In-and-Out Surgery Department, said, "No, not videotaped, but six nurses witnessed the fact that, without talking to the patients or examining them other than to introduce himself, Professor Querbol filled out the history and physical exam forms and went directly to performing the procedure."

CFO Slymowicz, with a side-glance to President Narrsey, replied in an ominous tone, "Those six nurses may not be available to talk to the NMCRB when they come to town next week."

Professor Querbol was aware of the other committee members' sidelong glances at him and the hushed whispering between them, and felt the need to say something even though he knew it would be summarily discounted. He had been appointed as department chair several years ago, coming from a position in a world famous east coast medical center, and his specialty training had been done in a highly regarded, nationally recognized program. In the NAMC's rush to hire him, they had acceded to his request to not seek information from his previous employers regarding his professional qualifications. As events played out, it was not surprising when a former associate later remarked to an NAMC physician, "Thank God you have that turkey. We thought we'd be stuck with him forever."

Professor Querbol now stood up to draw their attention, declaring, "The nurses are antagonistic to me and will say anything to harm my reputation."

The members did not comment, but looked stony-faced at the shifty-eyed Querbol as he sat down. The few times he had spoken in the past had been forgettable and uninformative. What the members did recall about Querbol was an incident in which the Medical Center Post Office had intercepted child pornography literature ordered by him at taxpayers' expense.

If that weren't enough, President Narrsey later admonished him for 'mistakenly' downloading electronic files of Nazi memorabilia from the internet into patients' charts. Since he was tenured, he could not easily be removed from his position as department chair. This matter had provoked a great deal of discussion among the faculty about what, if any, behavior could trump tenure and lead to sanctions and how far the administration would go to cover their own mistakes and proof of their bad hiring habits.

IV.

National Medical Center Review Board (NMCRB) Interview

Show me a liar and I'll show thee a thief.

~George Herbert

One week later

Much to the disappointment of the NMCRB team when they arrived, none of the personnel that had reported the 'ghost surgery' and falsification of medical records were available to answer questions.

Slymowicz was masterful in the way he managed the interview. He produced charts for all of Dr. Querbol's in-and-out surgery patients, demonstrating that histories and physicals had been recorded. Without contrary testimony from the nurses who were eyewitnesses to the falsification of records, all of whom had been immediately terminated from their positions upon suspicion of reporting unethical practices, the allegations were dismissed.

As for the 'ghost surgery' complaint, Slymowicz certified that while on his way to OR Number 22 to do the complex part of the case Querbol had started, MacBuckmaker had been called to the Emergency Department to give emergency care to a busload of hemophiliacs who had been involved in a motor vehicle accident. MacBuckmaker had in fact saved the lives of six of them by donating his own blood. As Slymowicz had promised, the review found no reason to sanction the NAMC. The team left without incident.

The NAMC leadership was appropriately grateful to Slymowicz, who was overheard to quip, "It's what we learn in law school: if the facts are on your side, use them. If not, lie."

11

Slymowicz, satisfied that he had pulled the fat out of the fire this time, then devised a plan that would ensure that nothing like this would occur in the future. When he requested permission to implement his proposal, President Narrsey glanced through it and remarked, "Ingenious!"

While a review board, which certifies their standard of care, must oversee every medical center the NMCRB was not the only such organization able to grant this certification. Attorney Slymowicz suggested that the NAMC affiliate with the North Kompliant Review Board (NKRB). Although it would cost twice the membership dues, he promised the hospital would never be in trouble again. It would be well worth the cost-- hardly one complex spine procedure. "Proceed in all haste!" was Narrsey's reply.

V.

Medical Complications Committee, NAMC

All animals are equal, but some animals are more equal than others.

~George Orwell

Three months later

Professor Williams opened the meeting with feedback from the Executive Committee regarding the five-times-expected mortality and morbidity rates for the complex spine surgery service and the high urinary tract infection rate.

After some discussion, the executive committee settled on the solution to the urinary tract infection rate. It was decided, with strong input from the President and the CFO, that this problem could be solved by terminating the practice of doing urine cultures to check for infection.

"That will give us a zero-infection rate and move us to the top of the list in that category," said Slymowicz, with evident satisfaction. Dr. Suum raised the possibility that a zero-infection rate might not stand scrutiny. President Narrsey assured them all that he could fix any questions that might arise.

It occurred to Dr. Nicodeum that this would also give Slymowicz the chance to reduce the institutional payroll by adding a few laboratory technicians to the parade of nurses that were dismissed prior to the NMCRB submitting their report.

"The complex spine surgery rates are more problematic, but the solutions should prove acceptable," said Williams. "Regarding mortality, many of the deaths are among the elderly and as such these patients have associated pathologies, such as coronary artery disease, renal failure, advanced pulmonary disease, hepatic failure, and advanced diabetes."

Dr. Suum interjected, "Because they are elderly, their spinal imaging studies all show changes that some complex spine surgeons consider indications for fusion."

"That aside," said Dr. Williams, rolling his eyes, "since these deaths usually occur within a few days after surgery, we can list the primary cause of death as myocardial infarction, renal failure, pulmonary failure, end stage hepatic decompensation, multiple organ failure, etc. I think you get the point."

"Do we ever," interrupted Dr. Suum. "But consider the consequences if this scam is ever uncovered!"

"Slymowicz has assured me that our certifying organization, the NKRB, is unlikely to give us problems," answered Narrsey.

"How can the solution to the spine surgery infection problem top that?" asked Dr. Suum.

"In many ways, it does," responded Williams. "As you know, all complications must be reported using a numeric code, including post-operative infections. Dr. MacBuckmaker has come up with the ingenious solution that instead of recording his procedure for treating wound infections in the customary way, such as incision and drainage, which carries a standard code, he will label the procedure 'spruce up', for which there is no code and therefore cannot be tabulated as an infection."

"Moving on," continued Dr. Williams, "we have two matters which some will insist pertain to ethical issues, and for that reason I've asked the entire medical ethics committee of the NAMC to join us today and participate in discussing these two cases."

"That will be refreshing," Dr. Suum cut in, "since we seem never to have had ethical problems arise in our discussions before."

Dr. Jones chimed in, "In fact, I don't remember ever discussing anything with ethical implications in this committee."

Looking at the ceiling, Dr. Williams asked Dr. R. R. Rad, chair of the Imaging Department, to present the next case. Dr. Rad stood up, walked to an X-ray view box and, while putting up four films, recited the patient's case history.

"An 8-year-old boy falls down and hits his head while playing with friends at home. No reported loss of consciousness and no marks of trauma noted on his head, although he does have a thick head of hair and a less-than-careful exam might miss marks of trauma. He resumes his normal activity, but after ten to fifteen minutes complains of a headache to his mother. When the headache worsens, she takes him to the pediatric emergency department at the University Hospital where he is examined by the house officers and the attending MD on call.

"Other than the headache, no objective signs of neurologic deficit are found, and he is given an analgesic and sent for a CT scan of the head. The scan is read by the resident as negative and so reported to the attending physician in the ED. When the child returns to the ED, he reports the headache has improved and he is sent home with medication and the usual head injury forms. Once home, he goes to bed where he is found dead the next morning."

Everyone in the room hoped that this tragic death had been unavoidable, but they all knew that the fact it was being presented to them suggested otherwise. Dr. Rad then reviewed the CT scan done at the hospital the night before the child died, pointing out a clearly visible cerebellar infarction, most likely due to a dissection of the vertebral artery. "How the resident missed this is inexplicable," he said.

"Isn't an attending radiologist supposed to be on call who could go over the CT scan with the resident, thus avoiding a preventable death like this?" asked one of the committee members.

"No, we don't require the attendings to be in the hospital at night," replied Dr. Rad. "The residents for the most part are almost as good as the attendings."

Verbalizing everyone's thoughts, another member replied, "Does that statement mean we have very exceptional residents, or very unexceptional attendings?"

Dr. Suum then asked, looking directly at Dr. Rad, "Why do you refer to the attendings as having to be in the hospital? All the other radiologists around the country can sit in bed at home and read the images on a laptop and report their findings to the ED."

With visible aggravation, Dr. Rad replied, "My attendings work hard enough during the day. They are not going to take night calls in any form as long as I am chairman!"

Clearly upset over this statement, Dr. Suum looked around the room at the other committee members. "Wouldn't you want, and even insist, that Dr. Excel, the well-respected neuroradiologist, read the CT scan if it were your 8-year-old son who was in this situation?"

All agreed, and Dr. Rad quickly changed his tune. "Under those circumstances, Dr. Excel would of course interpret the scan and do so willingly, but we cannot expect him to be on call routinely."

Dr. Suum, in disbelief at what he was hearing, posed the defining question to everyone in the room. "Are you saying there is one standard of care for those in this room, and another for the people on the street?"

No one disputed his statement, and Dr. Suum shook his head, appalled. Clearly the culture at the New Age Medical Center was much newer and more frightening than he had realized.

Dr. Williams moved on to present the second complication case. "Two weeks ago, a brain biopsy was performed on a patient suspected of having a low grade glioma. The pathology report was delayed, and in the interval the instruments used for the biopsy were sterilized in the routine fashion and used in another surgical case. The problem here is the biopsy came back positive for Creutzfeldt-Jakob disease, the infectious agent being a prion, which requires special sterilization to make the instruments safe for use in surgical procedures. There is a possibility that the patient operated on with the potentially contaminated instruments might develop Creutzfeldt-Jakob, a fatal, untreatable disease, but this is not certain.

"The question before us is, should the patient be informed of his risk of getting this disease, or should we say nothing? Slymowicz has already recommended we do nothing, because telling the patient would almost certainly invite a lawsuit."

Dr. Suum, unable to stifle his ethical concerns as the others apparently had done, tried one last time. "The patient has the right to know, and it is our duty to give him the information needed to make healthcare decisions in the future, such as should he look for further life insurance, or should he refrain from signing up as an organ donor. Not telling him of his possibility of an early death would be unethical on our part, and rob him of the opportunity to make informed decisions regarding his life going forward."

After a brief discussion, the committee voted to approve Slymowicz's recommendation and avoid any chance of an expensive lawsuit.

VI.

Executive Committee, NAMC

One month later

As the next executive committee meeting was coming to an end, President Narrsey informed the group that Dr. Suum was no longer on the committee and, in fact, had been relieved from participating in any further administrative committees.

"I am sure it has been as apparent to all of you as it has been to me that his persistent criticisms of our decisions call into question his loyalty to me and to this institution, and the goals we have set before us to achieve. In addition, I've instructed Professor Querbol to double Dr. Suum's teaching load, which will cut down on his operative time, which incidentally will decrease his income. Finally, I am transferring his stipend for student and resident teaching to Dr. MacBuckmaker. This will make it clear to him - and others - that there is a price to be paid for disloyalty to me and this administration."

VII.

President Narrsey's Large, Cherry Paneled Office

The most fluent talkers or most plausible reasoners are not always the justest thinkers.

~William Hazlitt

One Month Later

Smiling as he handed a glass of wine to Snow Queen, Narrsey sat down in an overstuffed red leather chair next to his favorite faculty member. He took a sip of wine from his glass. "Professor Querbol has just informed me that Dr. Suum has accepted a position at another medical center."

Snow Queen continued sipping her drink with a small smile on her lips. Her response captured what they had often shared in the past about Suum's contribution, or lack thereof, to Narrsey's goals for the NAMC. "These hinterland educated physicians with their hinterland values will always be problematic for us. Unfortunately, it's not possible to persuade as many of our type as we would wish to follow us to the north woods, where we can develop a record to further our climb into the medical hierarchy. We must be sure his replacement comes from east of the Alleghenies."

Nodding in agreement, Narrsey responded, "We've demonstrated that troublemakers can be squeezed out without incurring legal liability, a lesson I trust the rest of the faculty will take to heart."

19

VIII.

Commissioner's Office, Physicians Monitoring Committee (PMC)

While truth is always bitter, pleasantness waits upon evil doing.

~St. Jerome

Two months later

Dr. Jeckel, recently appointed commissioner of the Physician's Monitoring Committee, frowned as Attorney Ducus described a complaint recently filed with the PMC.

"This is potentially serious business for us," he said, emphasizing a fact that was immediately apparent to Dr. Jeckel. "The complaint is from a professor on the faculty of the NAMC, a former member of our committee, and when he reports professional misconduct, you can be sure he knows what he is talking about."

"What are the specifics of the complaint?" Dr. Jeckel asked.

" 'Ghost surgery' and falsification of medical records," replied Ducus.

"Is there any way this can be side-tracked?" Jeckel asked. "You're the lawyer. You must have some tricks up your sleeve."

Ducus replied, "I can think of several possibilities to shut this down, but if they backfire in a high profile case like this appears to be, the consequences could be disastrous."

"This comes at a bad time," said Jeckel, "I was just about to implement a program that would relieve some of the burdens I've seen our committees put on the physicians of this state in the past. Before I became commissioner, I had a leadership position in a major metropolitan hospital where I was continually aware of physicians who spent long years in

20

obtaining their medical training and doing what was necessary to build a successful professional practice only to be flagged down by the PMC for some minor infraction. It always took a toll on the doctor and his family. It is not fair and I intend to correct the situation."

Ducus, well aware of the laws in place to monitor the state physicians, could only wonder what was on the commissioner's mind.

"Taking a cue from the Feds," continued Jeckel, "I plan to develop a Physician Protection Program modeled after the Witness Protection Program."

Ducus was barely able to keep a straight face as he contemplated the problems in developing such a hare-brained scheme, so far outside the current legal foundations of the Health Department.

"The fact that our budget is being cut only makes it easier," Jeckel went on, "because we can't afford to have as many hearings as we did in the past. If we can settle complaints before the hearing process by offering the physician a slap on the wrist for regular types of infractions and relocating physicians with serious complaints to another hospital on the other side of the state, the profession will be well served, in my opinion."

"Very true," replied Ducus, still not believing what he was hearing, "but this complaint from the NAMC comes from a physician who knows both the NAMC and the PMC inside out and he has dotted all the 'i's and crossed all the 't's'."

"Think of something!" ordered the Commissioner. "That is what we are paying you for."

Ducus rose from his chair and started to leave the office, then stopped and turned back toward the Commissioner. "There is some risk to it, but we've used it in the past when the press has been fussy about one of our decisions or accused us of a failure to act on various physician problems that garnered public interest. The laws we operate under specifically protect the facts developed in our investigations. If we don't use them in a hearing, or if we give only selective facts to the committee that decides whether a hearing should be held thus ensuring there will be no hearing, the matter can be buried forever."

Ducus paused, and then added with a worried look on his face, "Of course, if one of the investigators in the regional office goes to the press, this would blow up in our face."

Jeckel, without hesitation, said, "Go ahead with your plan. We'll have to accept the small risk involved."

Ducus nodded. "I'll send a letter to the complainant, who must be anonymous by law, asking him if he is sure he wants to go ahead with the complaint." Ducus opened the door to leave, recalling as he did so the phrase in the PMC's mission statement proclaiming that their primary duty was to 'protect the public'.

"Wait a minute!" called Jeckel, as Ducus was about to close the door. "I just remembered something that might be very helpful in this situation. I met President Narrsey of the NAMC about a month ago at one of the Governor's receptions. It was only briefly, as he was working the room like a politician running for office - reminded me of Clinton or Edwards. He didn't spend much time with me, probably because he didn't anticipate needing my help in the future. But he sure had the Board of Trustees and the head of the Education Department eating out of his hand like trained rodents. I thought at the time he saw himself destined for the big time, maybe even Washington, D.C. Now that I know what we are dealing with in this case, I'm sure President Narrsey and I will be able to settle this to our mutual profit and satisfaction."

IX.

Executive Committee, NAMC

By this leek, I will most horribly revenge.

~Shakespeare

One month later

President Narrsey burst into the room through the door from his large, cherry paneled office with a scowl on his face and glanced around at the gathering group. We've just been served with a lawsuit by Suum!"

Individual conversations ceased, no one wanting to draw the attention of the obviously inflamed president, but Dr. Nicodeum thought, "Good move, W. B., this will be fun!'

"The allegations were detailed and to the point. Dr. Suum claims he has been harassed, damaged financially and forced to seek employment elsewhere because he disagreed with NAMC administration regarding policies, which he alleges put the welfare of the public at risk. His attorney is claiming that these dangerous policies will be proven in court, and he is demanding a financial settlement for Dr. Suum."

Narrsey, furious and red faced, glared at the committee. "I'll see Suum dead before he gets a dime from this medical center!" he shouted.

Dr. Nicodeum, who was Professor of Psychiatry and a good friend of Dr. Suum's, decided she would start emailing W.B. about the crazy stuff now going on at the NAMC. Thus began an almost daily exchange between Drs. Nicodeum and Suum, such that Dr. Suum was privy to every remark and move the administration made regarding his case and what was being said around the medical center where errors continued to be swept under the rug. Eventually, Dr. Nicodeum would pay the price for her communication with Dr. Suum.

X.

Regional PMC Investigative Office

One month later

Ms. Delta, manager of the PMC Regional Investigative Office, was assembling her staff for a briefing. She waited until the coffee and sweet rolls were placed on the table, then passed out the letter she had received the previous afternoon from the Central PMC Office, commenting, "This is going to be a long, hot summer."

Eyebrows went up around the table as each member surveyed the letter. Fresh on their minds was the recent dust-up between President Narrsey and a national newspaper that had run a story about medical and ethical violations at the NAMC. There had been rebuttal letters to the paper and campus-wide meetings promoting Narrsey's viewpoint on the matter. The matter had then been dropped abruptly, amid rumors that Narrsey had important friends in Washington, D.C. who had shut the story down.

Ms. Delta explained that yesterday, after receiving this letter authorizing an investigation, she had called the complainant, Dr. O.O. Seven, to confirm his report and request his help in the investigation.

"He is a member of Drs. Querbol and MacBuckmaker's department and has promised to cooperate fully in the investigation. He will provide us with the names of other physicians and nurses who were eyewitnesses to and familiar with the events in the complaint. Also, he will get the names of the patients involved so we can request the appropriate charts, including the charts of patients who died after inappropriate surgery.

He assures me that the medical personnel will be happy that something is finally being done about this matter and will cooperate fully, but that the administration will obstruct us in every way possible."

XI.

Executive Committee, NAMC

Curses are like young chickens; they always come home to roost.

~Robert Southey

Two months later

President Narrsey was beside himself. He glared around the room while shuffling a pile of papers and mumbling incoherently. Gathering himself, he addressed the committee, who listened warily and uneasily.

"It seems that in addition to our present list of disasters going on around here, we are being investigated by the PMC," he said. "What's more, I've just been handed a request to submit dozens of charts to the local investigators and grant hospital personnel time off for interviews when they are called to the local office. It seems we aren't finished with the antics of Querbol and MacBuckmaker."

"If it's any consolation," piped up Slymowicz, "the money from the complex spine surgery continues to roll in."

"As usual, the best defense is a good offense and we will get rolling on that today," commented the President.

Narrsey was visibly transforming himself in front of the members' eyes from the out-of-control, ranting and raving individual who had entered the room to the controlled, self-confident, calculating person with whom they were so familiar.

"First, it's obvious that our enemies have a mole in our organization who is providing them with confidential information. Slymowicz, I want you to hire an investigative service to find the mole. Give them permission to use all means available, both legal and illegal, to do the job," said Narrsey. Turning to the Dean of the NAMC, he continued,

27

"D.B.L., here is the list of personnel that will be contacted by the investigators. I want you personally to talk with everyone of them and remind them that their employment at this institution, including their retirement plans, are in jeopardy if they cooperate in any way with the PMC investigators."

D.B.L. Zero had moved to America from Britain as a boy and considered his three first names a distinguishing feature. Most of the faculty considered the D.B.L. to be his only distinguishing feature.

Next, Narrsey moved around the table to the CEO of the NAMC, E.D. Shiftworkski.

"E.D., we are certain to get some bad publicity out of this and I want you to be prepared to respond to each and every story with a plausible answer that counters that story's facts. Remember, the facts are what we say they are! Repeat our version to the newspapers, T.V., and radio stations over and over again."

He turned back to the committee at large. "Finally, I'll personally approach the PMC Commissioner and see what can be done about this investigation. I recall meeting him at the Governor's reception last year, so I'm sure he will remember me. No one ever forgets me." He gave a sly grin. "Now, if there's no further business for today, let's all go into my large, cherry paneled office for wine and oatmeal raisin cookies. Professor Snow Queen was good enough to bring some foul smelling French cheese in for us today."

XII.

PMC Commissioner's Office

Something is rotten in the state of Denmark

~Shakespeare

Three months later

"The NAMC matter is even worse than I imagined," said Attorney Ducus, taking a seat in Dr. Jeckel's office. "but I've come up with a solution which probably will work, with your approval."

"Continue," encouraged Dr. Jeckel.

"The regional office has been busy all summer collecting evidence from patient charts and conducting interviews with nurses and physicians. Some nurses who plan to retire in the next year or so will not be available to testify at a hearing until after they retire, but we should be able to avoid a hearing entirely if my plan works."

"The crucial aspect of how this is resolved in our best interest is to keep the facts of this rolling disaster at NAMC out of the public eye," Jeckel interrupted.

"Exactly," Ducus responded. "As a result of the investigation, we obtained two different versions of the 'ghost surgery' charge. Numerous eyewitnesses, nurses and physicians, many of whom were in the room, confirmed the events reported by the complaint. However, Dr. Shiftworkski, CEO of the NAMC, gave the administration's version of the events, which I personally think sounds very reasonable."

"I am all ears," said Jeckel.

"Briefly, Dr. MacBuckmaker was delayed in getting to the OR by an emergency which required immediate action on his part to save the lives of a number of accident victims. In fact, he accomplished this by risking his own life in a manner that can only be described as above and beyond the call of duty. To his credit, Dr. Querbol watched the resident complete the operation with only minor complications."

"Remind me to travel the long way whenever I drive north in the future," Jeckel said, rolling his eyes and placing his right palm to his forehead.

"As for the charge of falsification of records, I think we should accept the administration's claim that without video confirmation, it would be unfair to impugn Dr. Querbol's outstanding reputation."

"You've done your work well, Ducus," Dr. Jeckel said thoughtfully. "President Narrsey has been in communication with me for some time now and I'll be able to tell him the situation is under control."

"But you haven't heard the best part yet!" exclaimed Ducus, "The law requires that we have an outside expert review our findings. If the expert finds no deviation from medical standards, there is no need for a hearing! We have a North Korean complex spine surgeon willing to fly over and review our findings, and I've instructed the regional office to show him only the administration's version of the cases."

"Brilliant!" shouted Jeckel. "I think we are about to put this baby to bed."

XIII.

President Narrsey's Large, Cherry Paneled Office, NAMC

A bad beginning makes a bad ending.

~Euripides

One week later

President Narrsey, Professor Snow Queen, Dean DBL Zero, CFO Slymowicz, and CEO Shiftworkski gathered around a mahogany table, upon which were several decanters of wine, piles of cookies and French cheeses, laughing at Narrsey's jokes.

"By the way," exclaimed Narrsey with an air of satisfaction, "I talked with the commissioner yesterday and I believe I have the PMC right where I want them!"

XIV.

Spine Surgery Office, NAMC

Don't count your chickens before they are hatched

~Aesop

One week later

Doctors MacBuckmaker and Querbol were laughing and joking while waving a letter in front of the other attendings they had called into the conference room.

"Look at this!" shouted MacBuckmaker. "The PMC has found that there is no evidence of misconduct after investigating our cases! I am sending a letter out to all of the medical staff and I'm going to call my malpractice attorney with the good news today!"

XV.

Office of Malpractice Attorney T. K. Boutique

The good have no need of an advocate.

~Phocion

One day later

Turning to his secretary as he hung up the phone, Attorney T. K. Boutique said, "Well, the good news is I don't have to defend Dr. MacBuckmaker before the PMC. The bad news is that it's an awful lot of money the firm won't get. Still," continuing his thought, "I've funded my retirement plan three times over and doubled the size of the firm defending him in court. Also, there are twenty cases waiting for trial and no doubt more will be coming in."

XVI.

Executive Committee, NAMC

There are moments when everything goes well; don't be frightened, it won't last.

~Jules Renard

One week later

President Narrsey entered the room beaming and humming a tune. He sat down at the head of the table around which the others were gathered.

"We hit the jackpot yesterday!" he exclaimed. "The PMC cleared our surgeons of any misconduct and the investigator uncovered the mole. It was Professor Nicodeum, believe it or not, who was leaking information to Dr. Suum. We actually scored twice with the investigation since the mysterious 'O.O.S.' who was mentioned frequently in her emails is none other than Professor O.O. Seven in Professor Querbol's department." He shook his head. "The degree of disloyalty to this institution and me is truly unbelievable."

By this time in his tenure, Narrsey had rubberized much of the collective spine of the NAMC's governing committees. The surface remarks of approval by members thinly disguised their deeper acknowledgment and appreciation that Seven and Nicodeum had done what needed to be done.

Narrsey continued, "The investigators and I met with Professor Nicodeum last night and I offered to give her a six month leave of absence with pay, during which time she could find another position, if in return she would disclose the names of all the faculty members who were disloyal and talked about me behind my back. She refused, so I fired her on the spot, packed her up, and escorted her out of the office. What will puzzle me forever, and what is so ironic about this situation, is that she has been recognized three times for her work in medical ethics by this state. I'll see that those awards are rescinded."

The committee was shocked into silence. Dr. Nicodeum was well known to all of them for her many years of outstanding service to the NAMC. But a substantial bimonthly paycheck was in jeopardy should anyone dare to criticize Narrsey's actions, of that they were well aware.

"As for Professor Seven, the situation is a little tricky. State law forbids retribution for making complaints to the PMC so care will be needed in the manner in which we get rid of him. Slymowicz, I'll trust you to study the by-laws and find a reason for us to fire him."

XVII.

Neurosurgery Clinic, NAMC

Any excuse will serve a tyrant.

~Aesop

One week later

Shortly thereafter, Professor O.O. Seven received a letter from Dean Zero informing him that his faculty appointment was being terminated based on an interpretation of Article 4, Section A, Sub-Section 3, Paragraph a, Sub-Section iib. The page of the by-laws carrying the relevant paragraph with the sub-section wording highlighted was included with the letter of termination. Dr. Seven was puzzled by how the wording highlighted in the by-laws could justify his termination, but he knew that the administration could interpret the by-laws any way they wanted to. The letter was copied to President Narrsey and CEO Shiftworkski.

Seven's incredulous call to the investigator after learning of the clearing of MacBuckmaker and Querbol's was answered with the expected, "The law protects all that information." Seven knew at once what his next course of action must be, and he disclosed it to colleagues after they finished reading his dismissal letter.

"The failure of the PMC to sanction MacBuckmaker and Querbol is a clear signal that the physician monitoring process at the central PMC office is horribly flawed. I'll test the PMC by reporting the NAMC administration for taking my faculty appointment away in retribution for reporting MacBuckmaker and Querbol for negligence and incompetence, which is against the law, as you know. Not only will I file a complaint, which by law they must investigate, but I am going to request they conduct a personal interview with me."

Dr. O.O. Seven was completely familiar with the laws governing the PMC, having served on their hearing process committee for twenty years. Termination of his faculty appointment was obviously retribution for his reporting of the professional misconduct of Drs. MacBuckmaker and Querbol to the PMC. He could recite the law by paragraph and section. The failure of the PMC to sanction the two surgeons, despite the copious data collected by the regional office, was a tip-off that the process had been horribly compromised at the central office, since the local investigators had been enthusiastic in the investigation and confident that it would result in punishment of the physicians involved.

Determined to see this medical catastrophe through to the final inning, Dr. O.O. Seven filed a complaint with the PMC accusing the administration of the NAMC, specifically President Narrsey, Dean Zero, CFO Slymowicz, and CEO Shiftworkski, of violating the law that prohibits retribution against a complainant for filing a complaint with the PMC. Additionally, he asked for a chance to talk directly with the commissioner at the central office.

XVIII.

PMC Central Office

Bringing owls to Athens...

~ Aristophanes

One month later

Attorney Ducus handed Dr. Seven's complaint and the accompanying request for a meeting at the central office to the Commissioner. Ducas said, "I'm sure the complaint will be easily handled, but the request for an interview is already a problem." The letter had been received in the usual way, meaning that many of the department staff had seen it before it arrived on Ducus' desk.

The contents had immediately spread until all who worked in the office knew them, a number of whom remembered Dr. Seven with great admiration and respect for his past dedicated service to the committee. Ducus, who had come later to his position, was aware of the strong feelings of his staff that Dr. Seven should be permitted his meeting, if nothing else, because it would be the fair thing to do. He had the strong impression that his staff would disrespect him if the request was not granted. He explained the situation to Jeckel, who told him to schedule a meeting with Dr. Seven, since they controlled the investigative process and the outcome was a foregone conclusion.

"And," Ducas added authoritatively, "investigate only Shiftworkski and leave the President, CFO, and Dean alone. After all, Dr. Seven needs to know who is running the PMC."

XIX.

President Narrsey's Large, Cherry Paneled Office, NAMC

The greatest griefs are those we cause ourselves.

~Sophocles

One month later

Narrsey, the Dean, CFO, and CEO sat in silence, each looking at his copy of the letter from the PMC informing the NAMC that Dr. Shiftworkski would be investigated to determine whether Dr. Seven's termination from the faculty had been retribution for his reporting MacBuckmaker and Querbol to the PMC for professional misconduct.

Slymowicz pointed out that the administration was vulnerable due to conflicting statements made at the time of the termination. "The official letter cited reasons dictated by the by-laws, while our response to the newspapers that reported the dismissal was that Dr. Seven had failed to cooperate in an investigation into the leaking of confidential information within the NAMC, and that he had shown gross disloyalty to the institution and its President," summarized Slymowicz.

"Well," said Narrsey, as he sipped his wine and nibbled on a piece of expensive French cheese, "we're still dealing with a cooperative PMC, but I'll make a note to email Commissioner Jeckel today to confirm we're all on the same page."

Dr. Shiftworkski seemed visibly relieved and thanked the president as he stood up to leave the large, cherry paneled office.

"It would seems," P.H. Narrsey said to no one in particular, "that Dr. O.O. Seven thinks he has a license to report."

39

XX.

PMC Central Office

You cannot teach a crab to walk straight.

~Aristophanes

Two weeks later

Dr. Seven had just left the office after a two hour meeting with Commissioner Jeckel and Attorney Ducus.

Jeckel looked over at Ducus. "I see what you mean when you suggested we give him an interview. It was like old home week the way he came through the office greeting and hugging the investigators and attorneys, and kissing the secretaries. Anyway, he's had his say and now we'll do what needs to be done with this complaint."

"We'll start the investigative process tomorrow," replied Ducus. "It will consist of interviewing Shiftworkski, finding no misconduct has been done, and issuing a letter clearing him of Seven's complaint in two or three weeks."

"Excellent," said Jeckel. "By the way," he added, "did you notice that after Dr. Seven had finished his summary of the problems, he made some none-too-subtle remarks suggesting I was complicit in the cover-up of this matter?"

"Indeed I did," replied Ducus, as the lines in the PMC's mission statement regarding its primary purpose of 'protecting of the public' crossed his mind once again.

XXI.

President Narrsey's Large, Cherry Paneled Office, NAMC

A cock has great influence on his own dunghill.

~Publilius Syrus

Three weeks later

The large, cherry paneled office, with its mahogany table laden with wine, single malt scotch, cookies, crackers, Dutch chocolate, Swiss and French cheeses, reverberated with laughter as P.H. Narrsey gleefully told the Dean, CFO and CEO that he had received a call from Commissioner Jeckel that morning saying that the letter clearing Dr. Shiftworkski and the NAMC would arrive tomorrow. Slymowicz was particularly jubilant as he pointed out the obvious success of his scheme for double booking complex spine cases, which was increasing revenue to the administration in a way that all could see, drink and taste.

The Dean cautiously noted that rumors concerning Dr. Mac Buckmaker's malpractice claims had grown in number to the point where local attorneys were thinking of starting a class action suit.

"No problem," responded Slymowicz. "MacBuckmaker has incorporated a business model, rather than a medical model, into his practice. Use of a business model actually is becoming the norm in all the high-income practices. As a result, Dr. MacBuckmaker is generating so much revenue that the five or ten percent of unsatisfactory results can be considered the cost of doing business and are easily covered by the increased revenue. This, of course, would not be practical with a medical model, which would require us to limit unsatisfactory results to as few as possible.

Besides, these surgical bad results create the need for many additional imaging procedures and laboratory tests during patients' prolonged hospitalization, all of which add to our financial bottom line. "No," Slymowicz confidently concluded, "make no mistake about it, we have found the goose that lays the golden eggs, in the form of our complex spinal surgery services. So, remember," he added, "if the local population appears to be walking around with a stiff looking spine, it's because, and never forget this, *fusion* changes everything."

Dr. Jones, who had entered the room in the middle of the conversation, was of the opinion that in addition to patients walking around with stiff spines, many were also sitting or lying down with stiff spines, out of work and needing narcotics to make them comfortable.

Dr. Williams, who had accompanied Dr. Jones to the meeting, joined in and asked Narrsey if he had heard the rumor that the Feds were going to investigate the NAMC for suspected Medicaid fraud. "The word is that Dr. MacBuckmaker was allegedly seeing fifty to sixty patients in a period of two hours at the Medicaid clinic, and after Dr. Seven had covered for him one day, he had calculated that after all the paperwork was done, less than five minutes remained to take the history and examine each patient." Dr. Williams paused, then added, "Not to mention that the business office was billing for a full hour of contact time with each patient."

At this, Narrsey blew his top and, in unrepeatable language, reviewed Dr. Seven's family history and where he would work after leaving NAMC – "No where! If I have anything to say about it!"

Narrsey finally calmed down after a few ounces of single malt and became suddenly very philosophical. "We have Dr. Suum's lawsuit to deal with and what looks like a Medicaid fraud investigation by the Feds. Rele, you and our lawyers will need to figure out a plan to pull us out of this."

Rele Slymowicz, feeling secure that his services would be required for years to come, responded with a smile, "I think we can bribe a judge or two; it goes on all the time, you know."

I swear by Asclepius and all that I hold dear, that according to my ability and judgment, I will keep this Oath and this contract.

To hold him who taught me this art equally dear to me as my parents, to be a partner in life with him and to fulfill his needs when required.

…to look upon his offspring as equals to my own siblings, and to teach them this art, if they wish to learn it.

I will impart a knowledge of the art to my own sons, and those of my teachers, and to students bound by this contact and have sworn this Oath to the law of medicine.

I will use those regimens which will benefit my patients according to my greatest ability and judgment, and I will do no harm or injustice to them.

I will not give a lethal drug to anyone if I am asked, nor will I advise such a plan.

In purity and according to divine law I will carry out my life and my art.

I will not use the knife, even upon those suffering from stones…

…but I will leave this to those who are trained in this craft.

Into whatever homes I go, I will enter them for the benefit of the sick.

Avoid any voluntary act of impropriety or corruption.

…Including the seduction of women or men, whether they are free men or slaves.

Whatever I see or hear in the lives of my patients, whether in connection with my professional practice or not, which ought not to be spoken of outside…

…I will keep secret, as considering all such things to be private.

So long as I maintain this Oath faithfully and without corruption, may it be granted to me to partake of life fully and the practice of my art, gaining the respect of all men for all time.

However, should I transgress this Oath and violate it, may the opposite be my fate.

~Hippocratic Oath

THE END

www.ingramcontent.com/pod-product-compliance
Lightning Source LLC
Chambersburg PA
CBHW071643170526
45166CB00003B/1415